NATA GROBBELAAR

MY FIRST PERIOD

Nurturing the Miraculous Gift of Hope and Promise as You Enter Womanhood

I humbly dedicate this book to the women who shared their love and wisdom with me and journeyed alongside me to build and strengthen me for life so that I could do the same for others.

To my daughters, Fallon, Rina and granddaughter, Elke, who constantly remind me that being a woman is beautiful, fun and infinitely precious.

Above all, I thank and love my Heavenly Father, Who in His infinite loving wisdom, formed me fearfully and wonderfully to be a woman filled with Hope and Life!

NeNaChCoCo

"We have a little sister,
And she has no breasts.
What shall we do for our sister
In the day when she is spoken for?

If she is a wall,
We will build upon her
A battlement of silver;
And if she is a door,
We will enclose her
With boards of cedar."

A Song of Solomon

Contents

I

MY FIRST PERIOD

YOUNG, FABULOUS, PRETTY

*Knowing that the women around you celebrate your
transition from girl to woman is an exceptional thing.
Womanhood does not announce the end of a carefree,
innocent and fun-loving
existence but rather the introduction of a whole community
of women with whom you now have deeper and more
meaningful connections.
This is your day!*

One

INTRODUCTION

This is by no means an academic little book. It is not meant to embarrass you but rather a conversation I would love every young girl to have with a loving "Mum figure" in their life before their first period.

I went through my first two periods without any preparation. To say my imagination went into overdrive trying to make sense of it all is an understatement. It left me feeling very insecure, anxious and ashamed. After many years of struggling with my self-image and confidence, especially around my periods, healing came in a very unexpected way.

In my early twenties, I heard a story told with such love, compassion and deep understanding that it changed everything for me. It brought a deep healing and awe into my heart that I never knew existed. That story is the reason I am having this conversation with you.

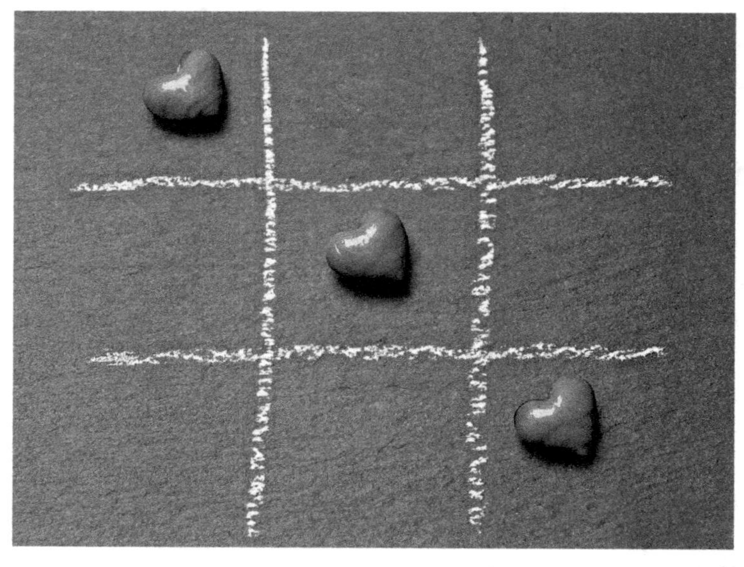

I was a medical student attending my placement in the Obstetrics and Gynecology department. Obstetrics is the specialty of looking after everything relating to having babies, and Gynecology is the specialty of caring for women's private health, like menstruation and breast health. I had the privilege of observing one of the most fantastic Obstetrician and Gynecologists I have ever encountered. What I learned from her has changed the way I look at myself and all women since.

One of the first things I noticed was that women find it hard to come to a doctor for any private issues, even if that doctor is a woman specializing in women's issues. Some were embarrassed, others anxious, and some hated that they needed to be there because it made them uncomfortable. Women's health is very personal and intimate, and it is hard to trust or ask anyone for help. It made me realize that, as women, we all feel the same.

One day, a young girl was brought in by her mum. She had her first few periods and was very anxious and struggling with understanding what was going on. Her amazing mum brought her daughter to have her questions answered because she did not have the answers herself. Here was lesson number two: Many women go through menstruation, never understanding exactly why it happens and how to navigate it. The story that the Gynecologist told them unexpectedly changed my life and started a healing process deep within me that I did not know I needed. This is the story she told with a gentle smile and soft voice:

"The uterus in your body has been waiting for many years to fulfill its created purpose. It is patient and needs many years to prepare. It has been given an essential purpose and holds many special gifts to do exactly what it was meant to do.

You see, the uterus is a small bag-shaped muscle, yet it carries hope and the promise of life. No other organ has such a great gift. It is now tiny, almost like your fist, but able to become as big as a watermelon when it fulfills its purpose and then returns to its original size.

The purpose of the uterus is to receive and carry a baby until it is born. To do so, it has to wait until your body is almost ready to have a baby. It then starts to prepare for a new life. Like a little nest, it starts building a warm, thick and safe inner layer, called the endometrium or the lining, and then it hopes an embryo (a fertilized egg) will come. While the lining is thick, it can protect, feed and nurture that embryo until a full-grown baby is born. With great care, it prepares every month, never giving up hope.

When no embryo enters it, it weeps and expels all the preparation - the lining falls out, and the raw uterus bleeds. It is not sad, though, because it is eternally filled with hope and the promise of life. So, the moment the nest is empty, it starts rebuilding. And that is the life cycle only you as a woman can carry. Your uterus is a miracle, and you have been chosen to hold it deep within you.

So when you bleed, it is not filthy, disgusting or shameful but reminds you that you are a hope and promise carrier."

Through the years, I've had this conversation, which I am writing to you now, numerous times with women of all ages. I have seen the beauty and self-love that come out of them when they grasp the miraculous gift of hope and the promise of LIFE they carry within them.

This little book is a gift from me to you: a woman, a sister, a mum and a grandmother. It is to you who are still innocently waiting for your first period, to you who have simply been going through your periods year after year without loving yourself, and to you who have got a young girl or woman in your life whom you are mentoring and preparing for life.

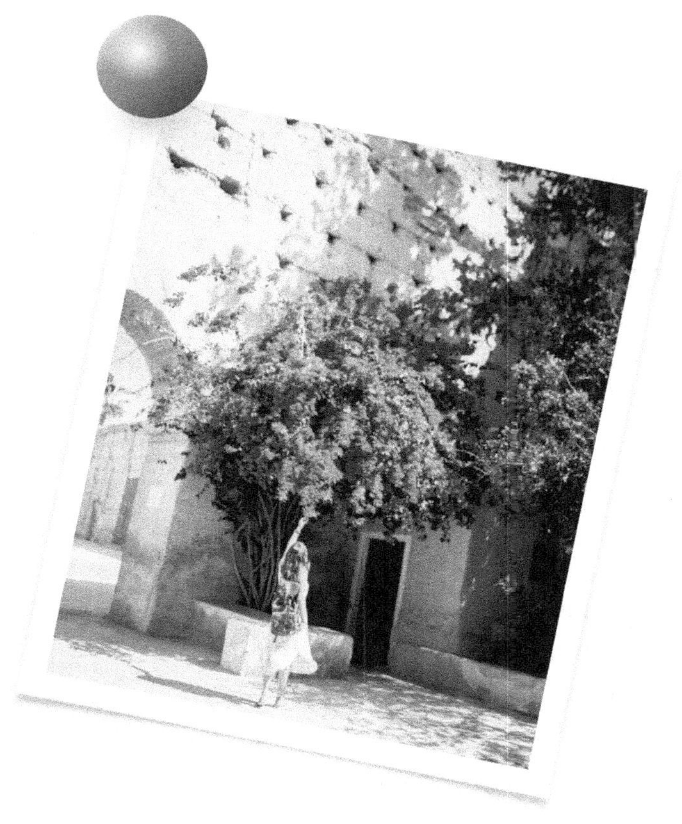

Two

THE MOST AMAZING PERIOD

MENSTRUATION - **That Big Word Nobody Talks About Openly.**

I grew up in a very conservative environment where some topics were either never talked about or extremely difficult to talk about. Menstruation or periods, the meaning and significance of it, was just one of them! I have a loving, caring mum whom I love with all my heart. Unfortunately, by the time she, with significant discomfort, attempted to tell me about my first period, I had already battled secretly with great shame and difficulty through my first two periods.

The fact is, I have come to understand in conversations with many women of all ages that it is not that women do not know how to initiate and have this conversation; Rather that they have very little understanding and factual knowledge of menstruation themselves.

Schools have, out of necessity, taken on this role. Although that is a good thing, no matter how well or clinically correct the topic is presented in a group setting, it cannot fulfill the inherent need of every young girl to hear about this very personal, sensitive and wonderful transition in their life from a loving, safe and trusted woman in person. Preferably a mum or mother figure who loves, empathizes, understands and personally supports her on her journey.

Each girl needs to hear the basics, but as each is so uniquely different, they also need the details relevant to her at the right time and place. As with myself and some other women, timing is crucial, and the window can be missed. I hope this little book finds you in your perfect moment.

WHAT IS MENSTRUATION?

Menstruation is the medically correct term for a "period." At a certain age, the uterus (or womb) starts shedding its inner lining (called the endometrium). It happens approximately once a month. The lining falls out, which leaves the inside of the uterus raw for a short while and causes it to bleed. The uterus is a magnificent organ that is the ultimate self-healer. Once the whole lining has fallen off, the bleeding decreases until it stops, and the lining starts growing again. Your female hormones regulate this cycle, and once it starts, it repeats throughout our lives until we reach our early fifties, when the process slowly stops, which we call menopause.

Menarche (pronounced men-ark) is when your period starts for the first time. You might have heard someone say: "It is the day a girl becomes a woman". Well, let's say it is the day your body is becoming mature enough to function fully like a woman. In other words, you are now capable of getting pregnant. It is a very significant event in a woman's life. Therefore, it is vital to understand the wonder of it. The promise of life is now a reality!

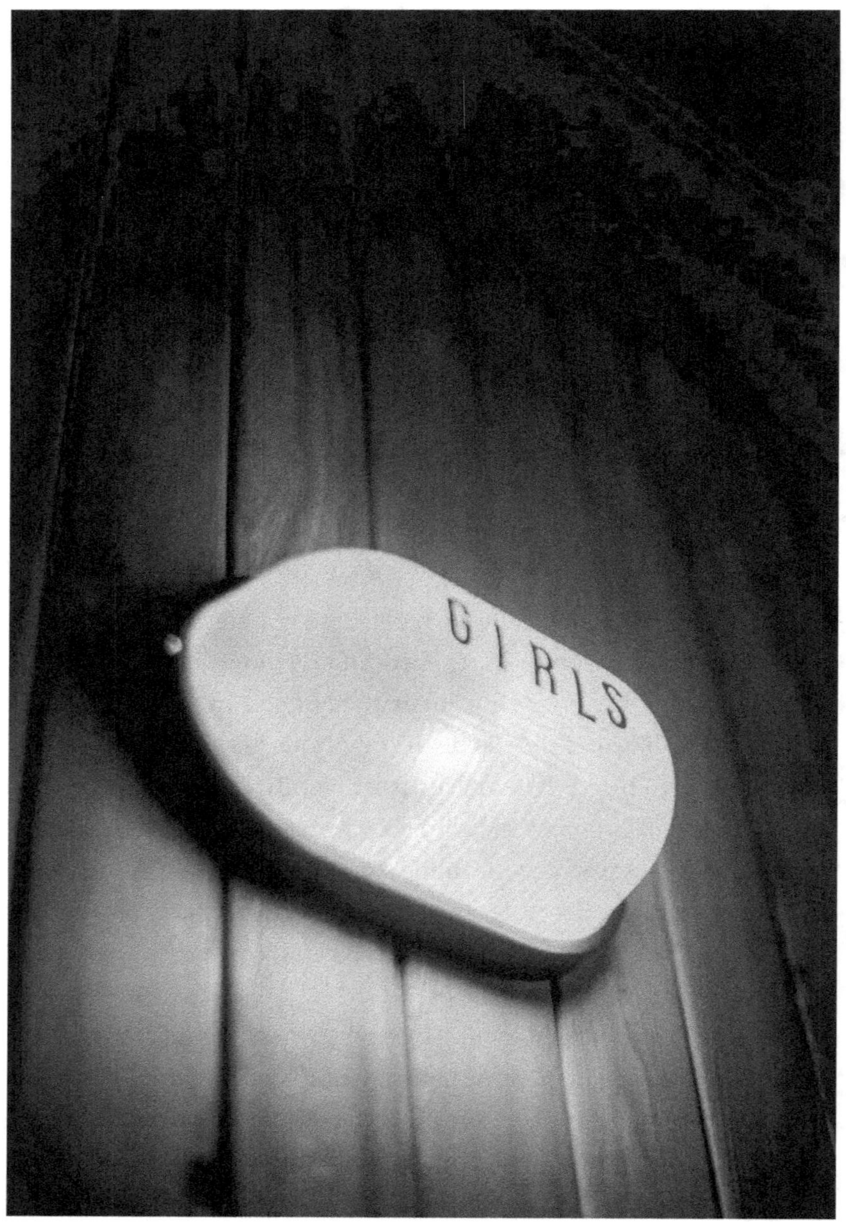
GIRLS

CONNECTING WITH YOUR MUM OR TRUSTED MOTHER FIGURE

It would be wonderful to have an open, loving and heartfelt conversation with your mum before your first period. It is a perfect time to connect at a new and deeper level with your mum or a trusted mother figure. If you read this, someone loves you enough to lock out for you. You are not supposed to be thinking about this stuff by yourself. You are supposed to love your life as a young, innocent, happy girl. And until now, that was enough.

I vividly remember that I did not give one moment of thought to a period, growing up or becoming a woman, until it simply happened to me. It is normal not to know anything about it. This is where moms, sisters, teachers or other trusted woman in your life come in.

As kids, we know that seeing blood is never a good thing, right? It usually means something is injured, broken or very wrong! It is not unexpected that if we have our first period and have not had proper preparation and explanation, our young minds come up with weird and wonderful interpretations. Some are very funny later in life, but can (as in my case) be very traumatic at the time.

I was at school when my first period started. I went to the toilet and noticed some blood on the toilet paper. I had no idea what was happening, it just felt very worrying. As the day went on, I took every moment to run to the toilet to check if I was OK. By the second day, the blooding increased. I was almost in a constant state of panic, fearing that the blood would show on my clothes. I bundled lots of toilet paper in my underpants and hoped to make it through the day. I somehow managed, and once I got home. I was far too ashamed and scared to tell my mum.

I do not even recall why I felt that way. I remembered that I once saw her buy sanitary pads, and when I asked about it, she said something like, "it is woman stuff". Somehow, I knew that that woman's stuff was what I needed and sneaked some out of her cupboard. My first period was a horrible experience of running to the toilet, not knowing what to do, what to expect, what to do with the pad…. My second period was not much better and left me with a deep sense of disgust and shame for myself every time my period would come along. The story I heard as a medical student changed how I felt about my period and how I felt about myself. The memory of those first two periods was no longer horrific but unfortunate. It also set me on a path to learn and help others to see what I now see - The beauty of a period.

I have a dear friend (now past menopause) who told me that she did not know what happened to her when she started seeing red come out of her and assumed it was the red cool-aid she drank. I never asked her if she drank it again. Hehehe…

Another young woman told me she had her first period before her mother planned to discuss it with her. When she saw blood running out of her, she assumed she had cancer and was too afraid to tell her mum about it.

I was told about a young girl who thought she had blood clots. We all have heard at some stage that having blood clots is bad. Imagine how fearful she was.

Many women will tell you what a blessed and wonderful experience their first period was. How their mum, friends and sisters celebrated the big event with them and how they were looking forward to their first period. This is the way I would love for all of us to be introduced to our first period, but things happen the way they happen. If this was not your experience, I can promise you (because it happened to me) that it is never too late to restore what was lost and broken and experience the same blessing and wonder.

Another lady told me that she thought she was bleeding because she went horse riding and injured herself. She was extremely distressed and scared to ride again.

A common theme I noticed is that many women felt too scared or ashamed to tell their mum or someone else that they had experienced bleeding. Many assumed they had done something wrong, and fearing what might happen to them kept them from asking for help. So you see, our innocent young imagination does not match reality when we do not understand what we are seeing, feeling and experiencing.

Perhaps you have already had a similar experience. It is NEVER too late to reach out and talk to someone. You can start the conversation from your side. You do not need to wait for someone to tell you what you need to know. If not with your mum, then choose a woman whom you feel you could trust to talk to about periods. Someone who can answer as many questions as you might have. From experience, I know that talking about the things, shame, and fears we keep hidden deep inside us sets us free and empowers us to overcome them.

Your friends might be talking about their periods around the same time you are about to have your first period; it is great if you can talk to friends while remembering that they are also just learning, experiencing and trying to navigate these new changes to their bodies. It is great to have a trusted friend to share this moment with.

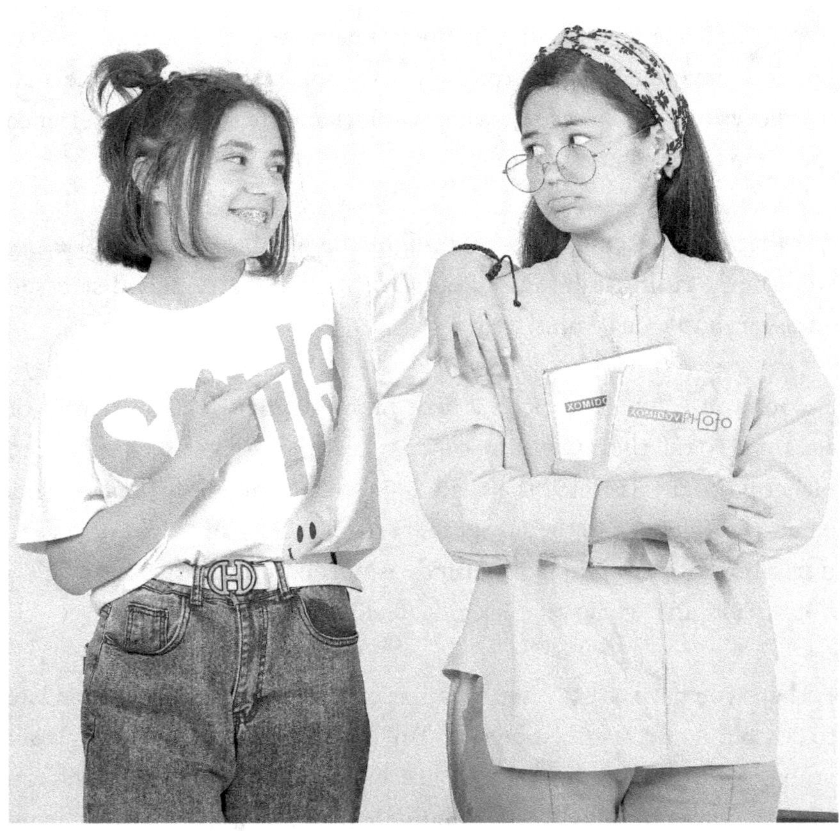

So, do not think for one moment you have to know everything beforehand. You have a lifetime to learn ahead of you. Your body knows what to do; you only need to trust and allow it, love it and be practical.

You might not know what to ask at this stage, so let's look at commonly asked questions.

Three

SO MANY QUESTIONS

Why Do Women Menstruate?

Female hormones, **estrogen** and **progesterone**, are responsible for preparing your body to become pregnant by the time you are an adult. These hormones cause your breasts to develop, the uterus lining to thicken, and the ovaries to mature and release an egg each period.

The hormone levels go up and down during the menstruation cycle. When the hormones are high, the lining of the uterus is thick and ready to receive a fertilized egg. If there is no fertilized egg, the hormones start to go down and cause the uterus lining to fall off and come out. That is when you bleed. That is your period.

Is it a Good or a Bad Thing To Have a Period?

Having periods is absolutely normal if you have a uterus. There is no reason to worry. The fact that you exist is proof that your mother started menstruating about the same age you are now as her body began to prepare to bring you into this life one day. Just think about that miracle for a moment. One day, when the time is right, you will answer this question for your daughter or a young girl who trusts you. It is a perfect thing!

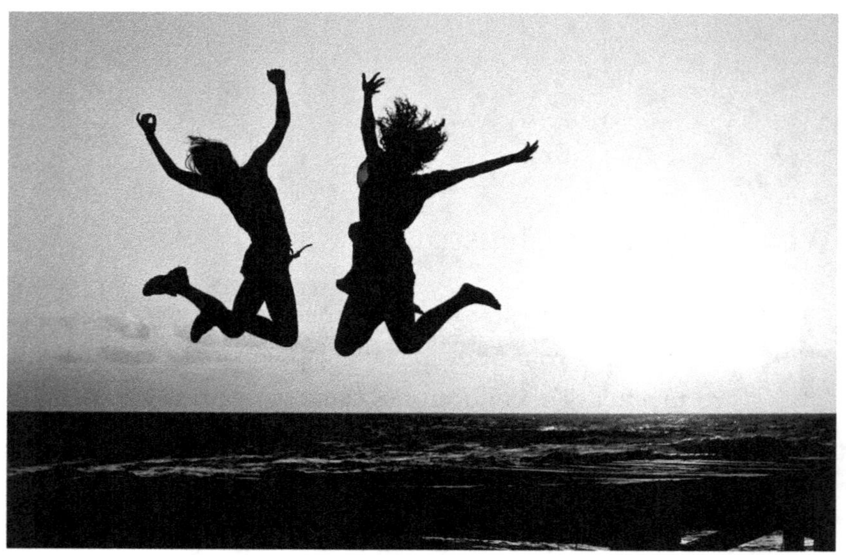

When Can I Expect My First Period?

Most girls will have menarche (start menstruating) between 11 and 14 years of age. It can, however, in fewer instances, be as early as nine years and as late as 15 years. Look out for signs in your body that you are preparing for your first period.

The first few periods might be minimal and vary in length. Your first period can be anything from 2 to 7 days and vary from spotting (small pink drops in your underwear or on the pad), a spot of brown on the pad or even red blood covering the pad. When you see red blood, it is called a flow of blood.

The best is to have extra pads available and replace them when the pad becomes wet. Pads are hyper-absorbent, so it takes quite a lot of blood to leave the pad wet. If you feel anxious, replace the pad sooner rather than later. By your second or third period, things will get easier!

How Can I Know My First Period Is Close?

One of the first signs that your body is ready for your first period is changes to your nipples. Initially, they might become slightly more prominent with a small lump of normal breast tissue behind them. Your first period will follow about 2-3 years after breast lumps appear—no need to worry if they are not identical. Normal breasts are not identical. One breast can even start to develop months before the other.

Few pubic hairs will start growing. (Under-arm hair only starts growing around your first period).

Your body shape will start changing. As your hormones increase, the position of fat deposits will change. You will become softer and rounder in some areas and remain the same in others.

A growth spurt usually indicates that your period is not far away. Expect your period within 6 to 12 months.

The fluid/mucous from your vagina will change around the time your breast lumps start developing. You might find a thin, wet line in your underpants at times. Around 6 to 12 months before your period, the fluid /mucous might get thicker and leave a slightly white line in your underwear.

What Are Some Signs That My Period Will Begin Soon?

These are some of the signs that your period is about to start. You might have none or a combination of these, and they may vary from month to month.

- Back cramps or stiffness
- Breast tenderness
- Headaches
- Acne or pimple breakouts
- Disturbed sleep pattern
- Mood swings
- Bloating
- Loose or more regular stools (usually a day or two before your period starts).

How Often Will I Have a Period?

How often you have your period depends on the length of your menstruation cycle. A normal cycle can vary from 26 to 35 days. The average is 28 days.

Should I Worry That Blood Will Come On My Clothes?

There is no reason to worry about that. Many women only realize their period is about to start when they go to the toilet and notice spotting in their underwear. There are different ways to keep blood from your clothes: sanitary pads, tampons, period underwear and period swimwear. Being prepared with a pad and extra underwear in your bag will set your mind at ease.

How Long Does a Period Last?

Your first few periods might be anything from 2 to 7 days. Being prepared for seven days is an excellent idea so that you do not find yourself feeling overwhelmed.

How Much Will I Bleed?

Every period can vary a little in length and amount of bleeding. The amount you will bleed is impossible to predict. Your first periods tend to be lighter than those that will follow later, but there are always exceptions.

You will not lose "too much blood" even though it might look like a lot. Our bodies are fully equipped to restrict and replace any blood we lose due to menstruation.

If you ever feeling faint or weak, it is normally not a sign of too much blood loss but rather the anxiety and feelings of being overwhelmed by what is happening to your body. It is not common, but when we recognize those feelings, we can self-help by knowing that what is happening is new but normal. Simply talking to your mum or support person will help.

What is a Cycle?

The menstruation cycle is the amount of days between two periods. Count how many days there are from Day 1 of the first cycle to Day 1 of the next cycle. Day 1 is the first day that you have a flow of blood. Sometimes, there is "spotting" before the first day. These days are not counted.

A cycle can vary from 26 to 32 days. It can vary a little from cycle to cycle depending on various factors influencing it. In the first few years of menstruation, the cycle might be closer to the long range.

What Influences My Cycle Length?

It is not unusual for your cycles to be a little irregular in the first few years. Keeping a tracker helps you to predict when to expect your period. As long as it is within 27 to 35 days and the odd, very long (up to 42 days) cycle seldom comes along, you are OK! If very irregular periods persist after three years, you might want to seek medical advice.

Things that will affect your cycle length are heavy exercise, eating too few calories, being underweight or overweight and certain prescribed medicines.

What Does It Feel Like To Have a Period?

It feels surprisingly normal. You will not even feel spotting. You will only notice it on your underwear or the toilet paper when you go to the toilet. When blood starts flowing, it feels like warm water running out. It does not run out all the time. Often, when we sit, the gentle flow of blood is held up; once you get up, you might feel a warm flow. As long as you have a pad in place, you will be perfectly fine. If you use a tampon, you will feel nothing.

As we are taught from a very young age to prevent urine from simply running out, it is a bit uncomfortable to feel you cannot control fluid running out of your body. That is normal. You will quickly learn to recognize how much you are bleeding and how to manage it.

Will It Be Painful?

There is no rule here. Sometimes, menstruation causes cramping of various intensities during your period and other times, it does not. Some women never have cramps, while others have them during every period. If you ever had sore muscles after exercise, you already have a fair idea of what cramps might feel like.

Pain cannot be predicted, but it can be managed and treated if necessary. It is essential to know that it is a normal occurrence and that there is nothing wrong when you do have cramps.

Some woman has cramps around the middle of their cycle when they ovulate. That is also normal.

Here are practical things you could consider if you have cramps:

- Drink more water
- Reduce fatty and sugary foods to reduce bloating
- Apply a heat pack to your lower back or abdomen
- Regular exercise to increase endorphins

- Eat healthy foods - You might include anti-inflammatory supplements (Vit D, Vit E, Magnesium, Omega - 3)
- Reduce stress

Can I Still Do Sport, Go Swimming And Go Out With My Friends During My Period?

There is no activity you cannot do during your period. As long as you have the appropriate aid to manage your blood flow, you will be just fine. Some girls prefer not to swim, but that is a personal choice.

Swimming causes no harm and poses no danger while you have your period. Your responsibility is to contain the blood flow. Period-friendly, reusable swimwear is a great option, and you can enjoy your day on the beach.

Another option is to use a tampon. I am personally not an advocate of tampons for young girls having their first period. A tampon is a cotton-like device you place inside the vagina to absorb blood, while a pad is placed in your underwear. Have this discussion with your mum or trusted female adviser.

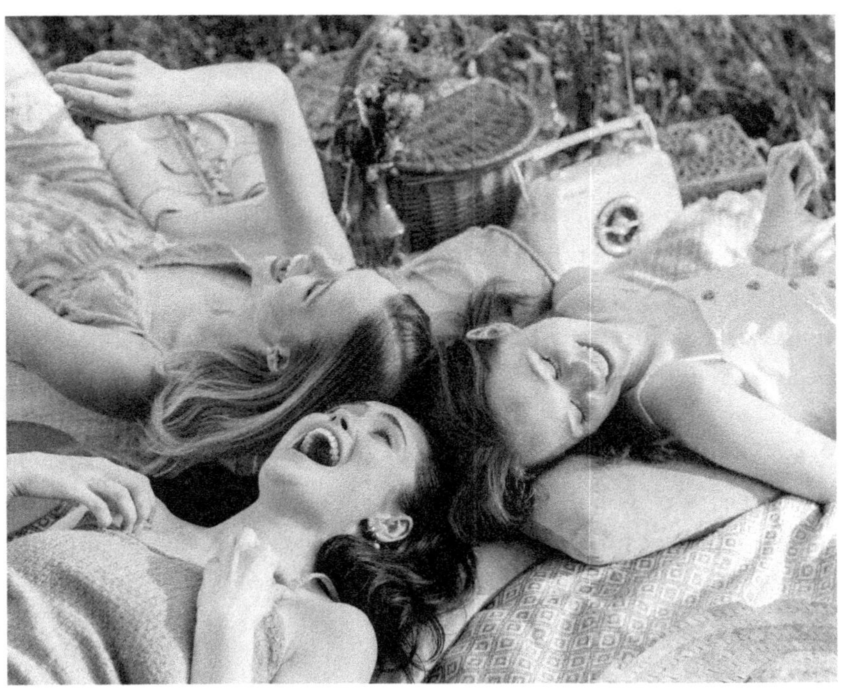

What Do I Do If My Period Starts At School And I Am Unprepared?

Many women only realize their period has started after going to the toilet and noticing spotting in their underwear or on the toilet paper. A hint that your period is near is when you notice slime/mucus in your underwear. As time passes, you will understand your body better and become better prepared.

Schools are prepared for such an event. All the female teachers can help you to get what you need. Schools usually have a medical bay where you can go there for help and advice. Schools should be well-equipped to help you without embarrassing you. If necessary, they can contact your parent to pick you up. Talk to your parent about your day and how it made you feel.

Your period is no reason to feel embarrassed or ashamed. All the women around you understand what is happening and will most likely be happy to help. We are all going through the same, and you would be surprised to see how easily woman band together when one of our "little ones" need us.

What Do I Do With a Used Pad or Tampon When I Go To The Toilet?

Most public and school toilets have sanitary bins in the toilet cubicle. Wrap the old pad or tampon in toilet paper and put it in the bin.

A pad or tampon cannot be flushed down the toilet as it blocks it up or does not flush down. We respect each other by disposing of the right way with period/sanitary products.

Wash your hands as you normally would when using the toilet.

How Often Should I Replace My Pad Or Tampon?

Pads should be replaced every 3 to 4 hours, as it can become smelly. Replace the pad quicker when you have heavy flow or do sport, and up to 4 hours with light flow and other times.

Tampons should be replaced no longer than 4 to 6 hours. For young women who choose to use tampons, use the smallest available and try not to exceed 4 hours.

Why Does It Sometimes Look Like 'Clots of Blood' Come Out?

The lining can look like a blood clot. It might be dark red/purple or brown on the pad or in the toilet. This is normal. The blood does not come out in clots but rather fills a pad or tampon or stains the toilet water red.

Does Everyone Have The Same Cycle? Should Mine Be The Same As My Friend's Periods?

No, everyone's period is unique. Your hormone levels, activity levels, stress levels and nutrition levels all affect your cycle.

Although we can definitely learn practical skills from each other, our menstruation cycles cannot be compared.

What Do I Do When My Periods And Cycles Are Irregular?

Do not worry about cycle lengths too much. You will soon see a pattern develop. A period tracker is helpful to follow your cycle. Be patient with yourself and let your uterus sort itself out. It takes a while to find its rhythm.

What Is Ovulation?

A female baby is born with about 1-2 million eggs in their ovaries. We cannot make new eggs but rather continuously lose eggs as we grow older. By the time a girl has her first period, only about 300,000 eggs remain. More than enough for the rest of your life. How amazing is that?

Ovulation is when one of the ovaries releases an egg. It generally happens in the middle of your cycle, about two weeks before the start of your period.

You might notice a slight tenderness in your breasts, an increase in the slime/mucus from your vagina and sometimes a little pelvic cramping or lower back pain. Most women do not notice these changes unless they are looking for them.

Does This Mean I will have a baby?

In the first few years of menstruation, it can be normal for your period to be longer and even skip a month. That does not mean you are pregnant. Only a fertilized egg can form a baby. That is a topic for later.

Four

PRACTICAL SELF-CARE

Dealing With Smells

Bleeding and other excretions from your vagina can become a bit smelly if you leave it too long. The best way to deal with smells is to clean yourself and replace your pad/tampon frequently. It is a good idea to have extra clean underwear available during your period or when you are more active than normal.

Shower at least in the morning and evening. There is no need to wash differently than normal. The vagina is self-cleaning. Using soap and rubbing can cause problems. What you have been doing so far is what you will be doing when you have your period, just a bit more frequently. You might need to shower after sport or physical activity as it can enhance body smell.

Face and Skin Care

The same hormones responsible for your periods also affect your skin. Changes to your skin can be anything from dryness to oiliness, a few pimples to acne. Every person's skin reacts differently. The best advice is to wait and see how your skin is affected and then adjust your skincare. There are many effective products to deal with acne. Make this your new daily routine until you reach an age where your hormones settle.

Acne can appear on your face, forehead, chest, upper back and shoulders and might have different appearances:

- Whiteheads and Blackheads
- Small red, tender bumps
- Pimples with white tips
- Large, solid, painful lumps under the skin
- Painful, pus-filled lumps under the skin

Most importantly, it is essential to avoid pressing, scratching and pinching pimples as it might cause skin damage, inflammation and scarring. If your pimples become infected, red and swollen pimples, you can consider consulting a doctor for treatment.

Five

LOVING YOURSELF

Choose To Love The Promise You Carry Within You

Loving yourself means you love every part that makes you so perfectly, wonderfully and uniquely you. The secret to being a loving human being is to love yourself first and then love others in the same way. As a woman, you are miraculously equipped to love much, nurture and mentor. Take some time to think about that…practice loving who you are, loving your body, loving your gifts and then look for the same uniqueness in the girls and women around you. The more we recognize these things in ourselves and others, the more we grow in love and compassion.

As women, we are so blessed to have a uterus. Remember the story that changed my life?

Let's summarize the wonderful lessons your uterus teaches:

- You can receive, grow, protect and nurture new life.
- You get a monthly reminder that giving up is never an option.
- You are constantly prepared for something new.
- You break down and build up again. You lose, and you. You cry and laugh…and that is LIFE!
- The more you repeat the same thing, the better you get at it.
- There is always hope; never give it up!
- It is through hope that you will eventually see new life and the fulfilment of the promises you were born with.
- You are uniquely and perfectly restored each time you fall.
- You are fabulous and pretty because you are a woman.
- You belong to a group of humans (women) who have a beautiful, unspoken, miraculous bond.

Your only responsibility, as you transition from girl to woman, is to love your life, live your dreams and enjoy every moment of it. There is no shame in being you!

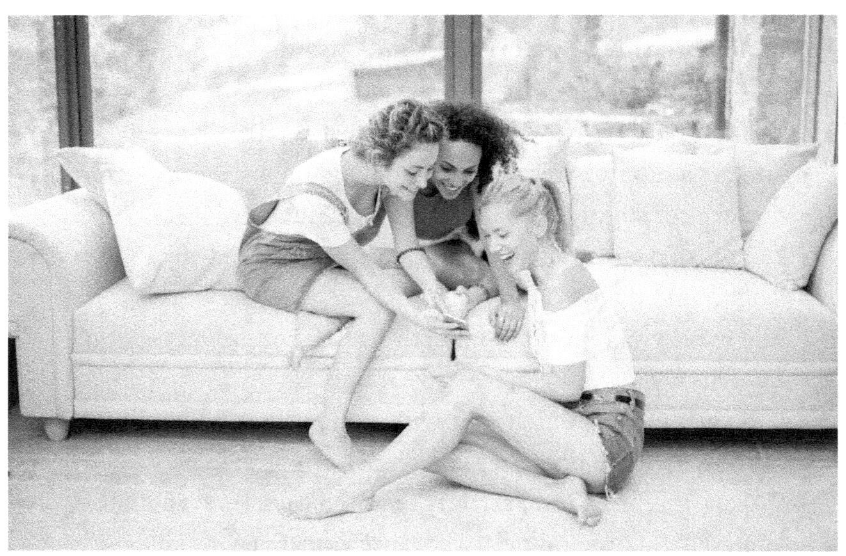

Choose To Love The Changes Your Body is Going Through

Your female hormones shape your beautiful body, soften your skin, restrict excessive hair growth and constantly regulate your maturing process.

The change in your hormones can cause your emotions to go on a roller coaster ride, but they also equip you to love much, cry and laugh much. Your hormones make you feel alive, and that is wonderful! Feel life every day. Please share it with your close friends and family, and make every moment count.

Every time a period comes along, I hope you remember that you are here because another woman - your mum - went through the same process you are going through right now. You are the promise she was born with. You are never alone on this journey.

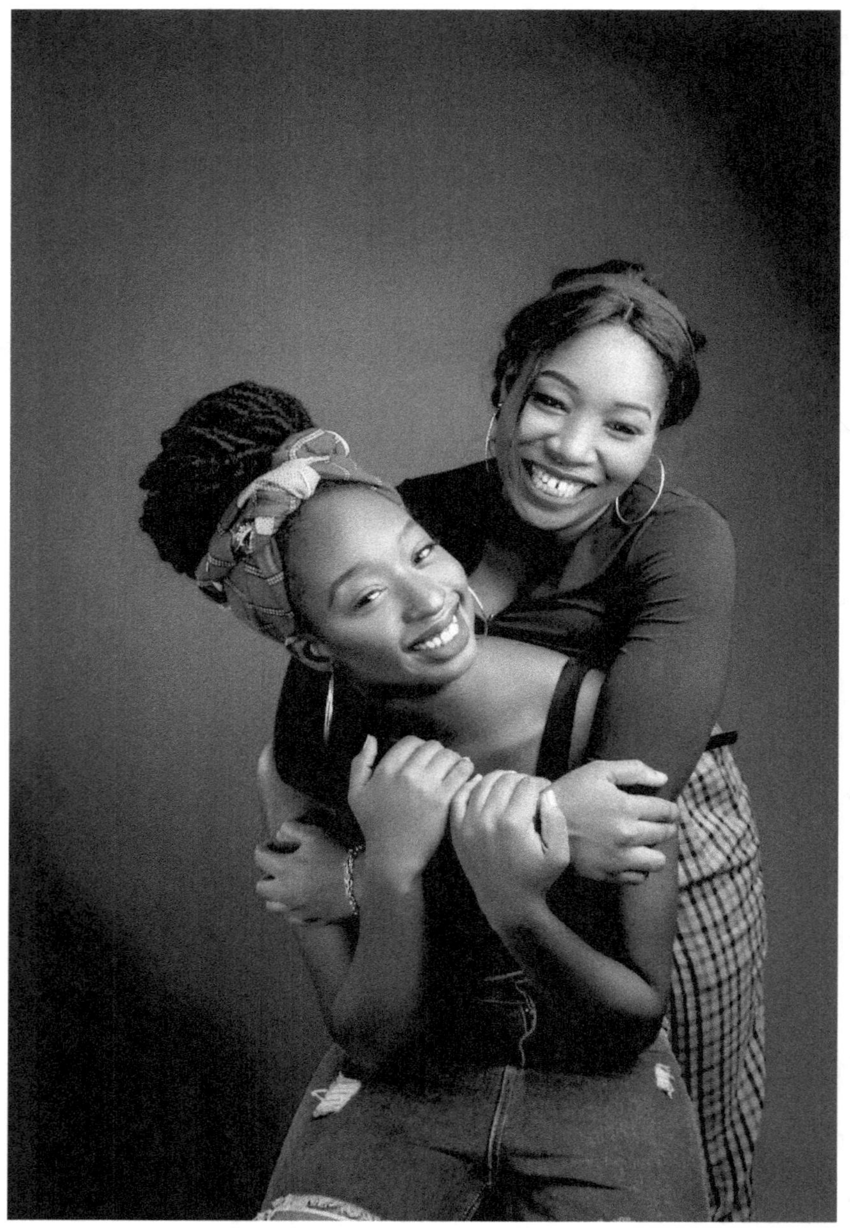

II

BONUS

We all experience anxiety, fear and stress when we feel out of control. One way of restoring and strengthening your feeling of self-control of your body is to be aware and keep track of your menstrual cycle.

This is a simple tool for tracking your periods. Menstruation should in no way restrict you from living normally. As you fill in your tracker, you will become confident in what to expect from your body, how to prepare for your periods and how to plan your social life.

Six

PERIOD TRACKER

What Should I Write In My Tracker?

1. Day 1 is the starting date - when you see the first blood flow. Spotting does not count.
2. How heavy is the bleeding? (Give a number from 1 to 5 each day. 1 = spotting, 5 = heavy / soaked pads)
3. Your **period length** is the number of days you have bleeding.
4. Your **cycle length** is the number of days from Day 1 of one cycle to Day 1 of the next cycle.
5. Once you have the cycle length, you can roughly predict the start of your next period. Remember it will take a few periods to recognize a pattern.
6. Be creative to note cramps, mood swings, ovulation (if possible) and any unusual changes to your cycle.

For example

- C = Cramps
- H = Happy / Good
- L = Low feelings
- A = Anxious / Unsure
- B = Breakthrough Bleeding (bleeding at any time outside your period)

Month at-a-glance

Month: ___________

SUNDAY	MONDAY	TUESDAY	WEDNESDAY	THURSDAY	FRIDAY	SATURDAY

Month at-a-glance

Month: _______________

SUNDAY	MONDAY	TUESDAY	WEDNESDAY	THURSDAY	FRIDAY	SATURDAY

Month at-a-glance

Month: ______________________

SUNDAY	MONDAY	TUESDAY	WEDNESDAY	THURSDAY	FRIDAY	SATURDAY

Month at-a-glance

Month: _______________

SUNDAY	MONDAY	TUESDAY	WEDNESDAY	THURSDAY	FRIDAY	SATURDAY

Month at-a-glance

Month: _______________

SUNDAY	MONDAY	TUESDAY	WEDNESDAY	THURSDAY	FRIDAY	SATURDAY

Seven

Conclusion

Every girl is born to become a woman full of life and promise. The only one who knows your value is you! Your first period, and everyone that follows, is proof that you are meant for LIFE, for HOPE and a miraculous FUTURE.

Just like your small little uterus, safely tucked deep in your pelvis, patiently prepare for a much greater purpose, so you are meant for a magnificently fabulous life. Your first period is one of the most wonderful moments in your life.

I hope this book finds you before your most amazing period so that you can embrace and celebrate being a woman. For those who find it later, I hope it will give birth to a beautiful story of healing and life in you.

For the mum and older women who read this, I hope you will confidently prepare our next generation of women, "our little sisters", with great love, reminding them that they have been created to be carriers of hope and the promise of new life! Together, we have the privilege to build upon them "a battlement of silver" to be beautifully and confidently themselves and "enclose them with boards of cedar" to be strong when trials and tribulations come, fully equipped to stand and support themselves and others.

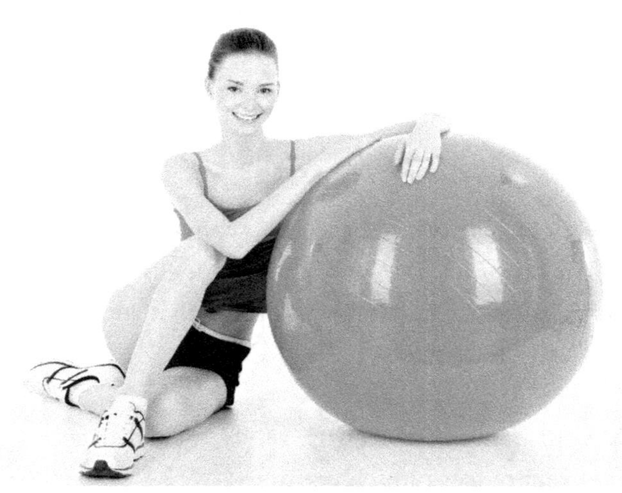

Afterword

Life is an awe-inspiring odyssey of constant revelation. Within each passing moment lies a reservoir of untold treasures and wondrous miracles waiting for us to unveil. As I embrace the profound purpose for which I was destined, my love for myself, life, and the pursuit of my dreams intensifies, propelling me toward the boundless fullness of existence.

This is my motto: "I live today by the choices I made yesterday, so choose wisely."

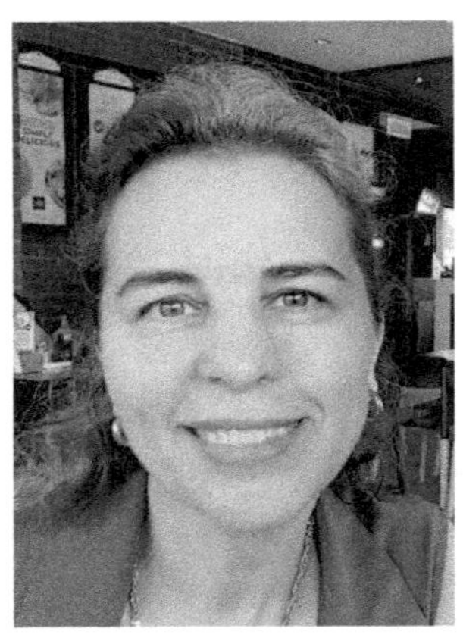

About the Author

Nata is a dedicated mum and mentor who champions the importance of self-confidence and self-worth among the younger generations.

With over a decade spent mentoring and guiding many other young women through transitions in life, Nata firmly believes in the transformative power of knowing and embracing your true self. Drawing from personal experiences, Nata has touched the lives of many young individuals.

Dedicated to equipping young girls with the tools they need to navigate and simplify the tumultuous years of adolescence, Nata has invested a lifetime of effort into targeting the challenges today's young people face and offering actionable and practical advice to overcome them. One challenge for young girls is seeing and celebrating the beautiful transition into womanhood without feeling overwhelmed, alone or ashamed.

Nata's vision is to light the path for the next generation, ensuring that every young girl realises their immense potential and inherent worth. The warmth, empathy, and expertise evident in Nata's work established her as essential reading for young woman and their caregivers.